HEADACHES

Megan Gressor is a journalist with a special interest in health matters. She was a health reporter for *Family Circle* magazine for several years, and has worked in senior editorial positions for other leading publications, including *Reader's Digest, Woman's Day* and *Better Homes & Gardens*. She was inspired to write this book by the lack of easily understood and available information on the most common of all health afflictions – headaches.

One half of my head in a mathematical line from the top of my skull to the cleft of my jaw throbs and hammers and sizzles and bangs and swears while the other half – calm and collected – takes note of the agonies next door . . . Anyhow, it hurts awfully, feels like petrification in sections and makes one write abject drivel.

Rudyard Kipling,
writer and migraine sufferer

HEADACHES
Relief at Last

MEGAN GRESSOR

ROBINSON
London

Robinson Publishing Ltd
7 Kensington Church Court
London W8 4SP

First published in Great Britain by Robinson Publishing Ltd 1995

Published in Australia by Gore & Osment Publications Pty Ltd

ISBN 1-85487-391-1

A copy of the British Library Cataloguing in Publication Data is available from the British Library

Note
This book is not a substitute for your doctor's or health professional's advice, and the publishers and author cannot accept liability for any injury or loss to any person acting or refraining from action as a result of the material in this book. Before commencing any health treatment, always consult your doctor.

Printed and bound in the EC

Contents

Introduction

Do you sometimes feel as though the top of your head is going to explode? Or that a tonne weight is pressing down on top of it? As though there's an army of elves trapped inside your skull, trying to drill their way out? Well, join the club. Headaches are the most common health problem – nine out of 10 women and seven out of 10 men suffer them regularly – and have caused untold misery throughout human history.

Headache sufferers are in good company – Frederick Chopin, Edgar Allen Poe, Alexander Pope, Karl Marx and Alfred Nobel were just a few of the distinguished victims of headache. This has led to the notion that headaches are a sign of intelligence or artistic talent. It's a nice idea, which has probably cheered millions of headache sufferers; they may be in pain, but at least it shows they're bright!

However, the sad fact is that headache strikes indiscriminately. A fortunate few have never had one in their lives, but the overwhelming majority of us are only too familiar with the distressing, and often quite debilitating, pain of headache.

What is a headache? A pain in the head, obviously, but it's not quite as simple as it sounds. There are many types of headaches, each with different symptoms, causes and treatments. There are tension headaches and migraines (the two commonest categories) and there are cluster headaches, neuralgic headaches, and headaches associated with eye strain, hormonal changes (menopause and the birth-control pill), allergies, hangovers and even sex. The pain can vary in severity, from a momentary nuisance to a pounding agony, lasting days, and victims have been known to bang their heads against the wall or even commit suicide to escape it.

The causes or triggers of headache are numerous, varying from something as simple as a change in the weather or eating ice-cream to serious conditions such as tumours. Fortunately, the overwhelming majority of headaches don't indicate any real health problems. While headache is, in fact, incurable – in most cases it's not a disease so much as a condition to which some individuals are more susceptible than others – appropriate treatment, coupled with careful attention to lifestyle, can reduce, control and even eliminate the pain.

This book is designed to help you identify your particular type of headache, what may be causing it, what medical treatment is available, how you can help yourself and what measures you can take to prevent future headaches ever starting.

Chapter I

If Pain Persists . . .

The vast majority of headaches are suffered in silence. In the belief that the pain will be short-lived, or that headache is one of those things that is sent to try us (and it does!), many people simply soldier on.

However, as they say in the advertisements for painkillers, if pain persists, you should consult your doctor. And not only if the pain is persistent; if headaches suddenly strike someone usually headache-free, or if the usual pain suffered changes in character or intensity, or is causing you any concern, it goes without saying that you should seek medical advice.

- **Consultation:** When you consult your GP, he or she will probably ask a series of questions designed to arrive at a diagnosis of the type of headache you're suffering from – whether it's an idiopathic ('precise cause unknown') headache, like a tension or migraine headache, or whether it could spring from some more sinister problem, such as a brain tumour or abscess.

The doctor is likely to ask where the pain strikes – front or back of the head? over the eye? – and how it feels – pounding or throbbing? a tight band around the head? He or she may inquire about any other symptom associated with the pain, such as nausea, vomiting, change in bowel habit or special sensitivity to bright lights, sounds or smells. And you may be asked whether the pain is increasing, whether it's worse in the morning or when you cough, bend or strain, and how it reacts to simple medication, like analgesics (painkillers). The doctor may also ask how the pain is affected by weekends, travel or other breaks in routine, and whether jarring the head makes it worse.

- **Examination:** The doctor will probably check your family medical history (heredity plays a part, particularly in migraines) as well as any medication you're taking for other conditions (headache can be a side effect of some medications which act by expanding the blood vessels, such as the nitrates used to treat heart disease). He or she may take your temperature and check your nose and ears for signs of infection – a common cause of headache – as well as check your reflexes and eyes for signs of neurological problems. If a cause for concern is found, it may be necessary to order blood tests, X-rays of your sinuses, a brain scan and/or refer you to a neurologist.

- Long before you've got to this point, however, you will probably have been asked about any personal problems or special stress you may be experiencing, because the overwhelming likelihood is that your trouble is a simple tension headache.

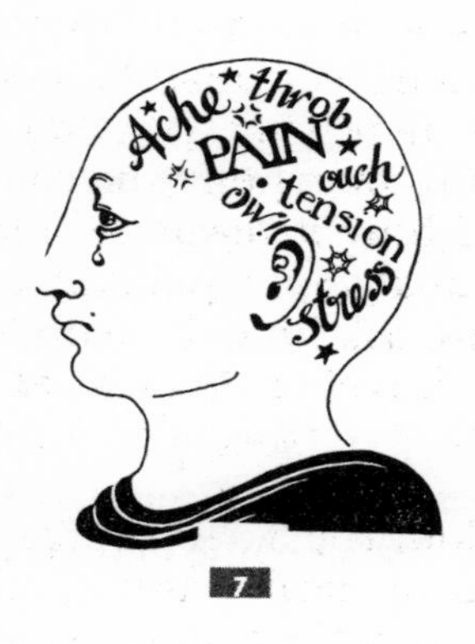

Chapter 2
Tension Headaches

'I was still suffering from the sick headache; but the instant I saw the contents of the note I was cured.'

– **General Ulysses Grant**, migraine sufferer and leader of the Union army during the American Civil War, on receiving word from General Robert E. Lee, leader of the Confederate army, that he was ready to surrender.

Your skull feels as though it's being squeezed in a vice. Your brains feel like they are boiling and about to burst out through your ears any minute now. Your temples are throbbing, your neck is a rigid column of pain and your shoulders feel so tight they could almost be in a plaster cast.

You are suffering from a tension headache, and it's probably no consolation to know that this is the most overwhelmingly common type of headache.

WHO GETS TENSION HEADACHES?

Ninety per cent of us endure tension headaches at some point in our lives, some almost continuously. They affect women two or three times more often than men. They can strike at any age: a child studying for exams is just as susceptible as a company director involved in a corporate takeover, depending on lifestyle and personality.

What is the Pain Like?

Sufferers often say they feel as though a heavy weight is bearing down on top of the head, and complain of a dull, constant ache pressing down and tightening around the skull. This can range from mild discomfort to a pain so severe it drives victims to beat their heads with their fists.

When Does it Strike?

These headaches often start in the middle of the day, afternoon or evening. They can last for several hours, sometimes days, and usually start at the back of the head or neck, moving forward to the eyes and temples until the entire 'hat band' of the crown is encompassed.

These headaches are also known as muscle contraction headaches, because the immediate physical source of the problem is often tension in the muscles of the shoulders, neck, jaw and

Typical pattern of tension-headache pain

(The darker the shaded area the more intense the pain)

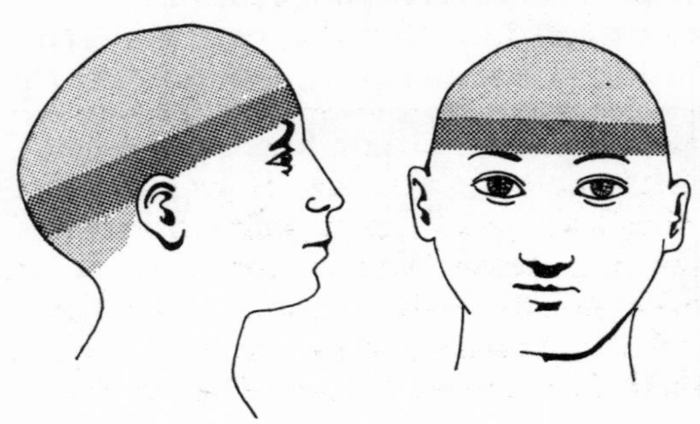

head. However, the root cause of tension headache is often (but not always) emotional. Before you can react appropriately to your tension headaches, you need to work out whether they are triggered by emotional stress or physical tension.

PHYSICAL CAUSES

The physical triggers of tension headaches are pretty easy to detect, and are largely the result of lifestyle and environmental factors. Our sedentary, but stressful, way of life is a prime culprit.

If you spend your working day hunched over a VDU in an air-conditioned office, fielding never-ending phone calls and forgetting to take a lunch-break, you are two-thirds of the way towards arriving home with a thumping headache. Poor posture is a major factor; working in the same position for hours on end causes postural stress and physical tension, whether

Aspirin reduces pain and fever by interfering with the body's production of prostaglandins – chemicals which cause inflammation and make the blood vessels contract. Brand names: Anadin, Askit, Aspro, Aspro Clear, Beecham's Powders, Bayer aspirin, Caprin, Disprin, Mrj Cullens, Fynnon, Phensic, Platet, Toptabs.
Aspirin with Codeine *(a painkilling narcotic)*: Codis 500, Cojene, Veganin.
Aspirin with Paracetamol: Actron, Anadin Extra, Disprin Extra, Nurse Sykes Powders, Powerin.
Paracetamol relieves moderate pain and reduces fever. It also inhibits the body's production of prostaglandins; however, paracetamol does not reduce inflammation. Brand names: Calpol infant, Disprin, Elkamol, Fanalgic, Hedex, Lemsip, Miradol, Night Nurse, Paldesic, Panadol, Paracets, Paraclear, Paramin, Resolve, Rimadol, Salzone, Tramil.
Paracetamol with Codeine: Boots Pain Relief Plus, Codamed, Codanin, E.P., Feminax, Flucaps, Migraleve, Panadiene, Panadol Ultra, Panerel, Paracodol, Propain, Solpadeine.

you're sitting typing at a desk or bent over a drafting board. Flickering fluorescent lights and the sounds, lights and fumes of office equipment, like photocopiers and faxes, don't help either, but many of us spend eight hours or more a day in such conditions.

MEDICAL TREATMENT

- **Analgesics** (painkillers) are the first line of defence for most headache sufferers, usually over-the-counter preparations containing aspirin or paracetamol.

  Such analgesics are usually effective, particularly if taken with the time-honoured combination of a cup of tea (or coffee) and a good lie down. The rest gives you a chance to relieve muscle tension, while the caffeine in tea or coffee can help contract dilated blood vessels (one cause of headache pain). These analgesics are reasonably safe, but be warned: overindulgence, particularly over a long period, may cause health problems. Aspirin can irritate the stomach and cause bleeding from the gut. People with peptic ulcers and bleeding disorders shouldn't use it, or should at least consult their doctor beforehand. Paracetamol is kinder to the stomach than aspirin; however, it can cause tummy upsets, and shouldn't be taken without medical consultation by people with peptic ulcers. It is also very dangerous to exceed the recommended daily dose. Both types of analgesic should be taken with a full glass of water or milk to protect the stomach.

If you consult your doctor about your tension headaches, you may be prescribed a course of **muscle relaxants** or **tranquillisers** to unlock tight muscles, or **anti-depressants** to combat the stress contributing to headache pain. Such drugs are also beneficial, but generally only in the short term. They all have side effects, and long-term use can lead to other problems.

Accordingly, the doctor is likely to recommend that you learn relaxation and stress management techniques, such as the ones outlined in Chapter 4.

Self-Help for Tension Headaches with Physical Causes

- **Posture:** Have a good look at the way you hold yourself. Are your shoulders slumped? Do you stand slouched, with all your weight on one foot? Is your head poking forward at an angle, or drooping down on your chest? When you sit, do you slump?

  If so, it's time to re-educate your body. It takes time to change the physical habits of a lifetime, but try to remember to stand straight, shoulders relaxed, with your head level and aligned with your body. Tuck in your chin. Your neck should feel long, straight and relaxed. Remember, always think tall!

- **At work:** Try to avoid sitting with your head bent for long periods of time. Don't slouch – your chair should support your back properly (typists' chairs are better than those lounge-style 'executive' chairs) – and try to rearrange your work station so that you're looking straight, not down, at your work (raise your VDU so that it's level with your eyes; pin paperwork to a clip-board, at right angles to your desk).

  Pace yourself – try not to work flat out, beating yourself into a frazzle to meet deadlines. Take a proper lunch break, and make time to go outside and take a few deep breaths of fresh air, even if only for a minute or two. Make sure that you stretch regularly and get up to walk around often.

  If your desk is below a flickering fluorescent light or next to a busy photocopier, ask to be moved or for something to be done about it. Avoid colleagues' cigarette smoke, wherever possible (this is easier nowadays, with many workplaces smoke-free zones), and go easy on the office coffee (more about caffeine's role in headaches in Chapter 8). If your workplace is very noisy, consider earplugs or discuss ways to reduce the sound (could the printer be enclosed in a soundproof box, for example, or put in a separate room?) Ask your union or workplace health and safety officer for suggestions and exercises to minimise work-related tension.

Poor posture is a major factor in tension headaches

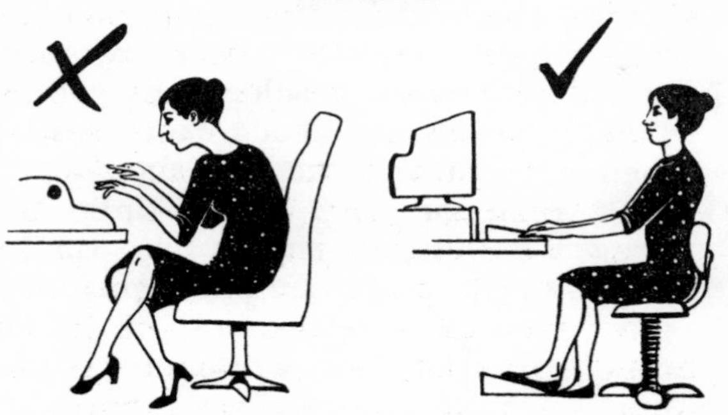

- **At home:** Physical stress isn't confined to the workplace, of course. A busy mother, picking up after noisy toddlers or mediating between quarrelsome adolescents, knows all about it. If you spend hours cleaning up after your family, only to have them return at the end of the day and wreck all your good work, you're a sitting duck for a humdinger of a headache. You, too, should allow time out for a stretch and a walk, a breath of fresh air and some time to yourself to relax and loosen up.

How to loosen up? Whether at home or at work, try to make time, at least once a day, to do these simple exercises:

Quick Stress-Busters

1. Sit with your arms held loosely at your sides and with hands resting limply in your lap. Both feet should be flat on the floor.

Now, breathe in through your nose for a count of five. Hold your breath for three counts, then exhale slowly through your mouth for five counts. Repeat three times.

2. Sitting in the same position, raise your left shoulder to meet your left ear, tensing all the muscles of your left arm, shoulder and neck. Hold for the count of three, then relax the muscles, letting the arm flop down. Repeat with the right arm. Perform this exercise three times, alternating shoulders, then repeat another three times, raising both shoulders together.
3. Position as before. Keeping your shoulders and neck relaxed, screw your face up as tightly as possible – frowning, tightening the jaw and screwing up the eyes. Hold this position for five counts, then relax. Repeat five times.
4. Position as before, remembering to keep your shoulders and neck relaxed. Slowly, turn your head to the right and hold for five counts, then turn it to the left and hold for five counts. Repeat this exercise five times.
5. Finally, stand up and gently shake out arm and neck muscles and have a good stretch before continuing your work.

EMOTIONAL CAUSES OF TENSION HEADACHES

It's all very well to do exercises to loosen you up, but you also have to work out what made you tense in the first place. While bad posture, poor work habits and the like are all contributing factors, the most common causes of physical tension are, in fact, emotional or psychological. These include:

- stress
- anxiety
- depression
- repressed anger
- fatigue
- feelings of guilt or inadequacy
- low self esteem
- loneliness
- fear
- pressure to perform and succeed.

All these can result in the physical tension that triggers headaches, and they arise from all manner of everyday events.

Money worries are almost universal, particularly in times of recession and high unemployment. Are you forever striving to meet deadlines and forgetting to take time out for yourself? Perhaps you're struggling to please an unreasonable boss, you don't like the work you do, or you've been passed over for promotion.

On the home front, you could be fuming because your spouse has disappointed you, a friend has let you down, your young son is having school hassles or your teenager is going through 'one of those stages'. Unrealistic expectations of ourselves or others, moving house, changing careers, sickness in the family – all these things take an emotional toll.

Self-Help for Tension Headaches with Emotional Causes

It's virtually impossible to alter the events that prompt such negative emotions, but learning to recognise when you are tense and identifying the emotional triggers are important, if you are to control the pain of tension headache. Once you know what is precipitating your headaches, you can work on modifying your reaction to it – and, with luck, avoid future pain.

If, for example, you always get a headache just before your overbearing mother-in-law comes to visit, your body is trying to tell you something about her effect on you. You can't change her, but you can change yourself and how you react to her. Are you tensing up because you fear her criticism of the way you keep house or raise the children? The solution isn't to whip yourself into a frenzy cleaning up before she comes, but to recognise that it's what you think about these matters that's important, not what anybody else thinks.

You're very vulnerable to negative emotions if you're low on self-esteem. So many of us have impossible ideals of what we could or should be doing – due, partly to media concentration on high achievers, superwomen and the like – and we tend to feel failures because we don't have wonderful jobs and love-lives, perfect homes and families, and look like Elle MacPherson, to boot. Well, don't look now, but there aren't too many of these paragons around outside the pages of popular fiction.

It may sound trite, but learning to love and accept yourself for what you are is essential to help build up your psychic reserves against the negative emotions that can lead to tension headaches. So, how do you build up self-esteem? Be your own best friend, not your worst critic. Tell yourself how terrific you are!

Try making these simple affirmations regularly, preferably every day.

- You may not be perfect, but you are a good and worthwhile person with your own special qualities and talents.
- You can't please everybody, so why whip yourself into a frenzy trying? Allow people to like and love you as you are.
- Remember that your partner, family and friends are not perfect either. Don't expect too much of them, and you won't feel let down.
- Don't suppress your feelings. Bottling up anger, disappointment and hurt will only make you tense and resentful. Speak your mind (choosing your words carefully, without being too harsh). Honesty is the best option, by far.
- Don't push yourself too hard at work. Do the best you can, as efficiently as possible, but don't take on too much. Learn to delegate, and expect from your work-mates as much as you expect from yourself.

- Don't torture yourself with guilt. We all make mistakes from time to time, and you can't change that. Come to terms with your failings – and failures – and learn to enjoy life, one day at a time.

Chapter 3

The Misery of Migraines

Migraine is the second most common type of headache, after tension headaches, afflicting an estimated one in every 20 people. Migraine pain can be intense, debilitating and, in some cases, can virtually disable its victims, putting them out of action for, generally, short periods of time.

WHO GETS MIGRAINES?

Migraine runs in families: around 60 per cent of victims will have a close relative who also suffers from migraine. If both parents are migraineurs (migraine sufferers), there is a very strong chance that you will inherit the condition.

Migraine can strike at any age. Children are not immune (see Chapter 9, 'Children's Headaches'), but it most commonly begins in the twenties or thirties, and starts to wane as sufferers hit their fifties. It's rare for migraine to commence in middle age or older. Since migraine typically strikes in the busiest and most taxing time of life – years filled with the hassles of holding down jobs, organising finances, starting families, establishing homes etc. – it's tempting to see stress as a major factor in the onset of migraine.

So are hormones. Women make up the overwhelming majority of migraine victims; eight or nine out of every 10 migraineurs are female. The female hormone oestrogen is the culprit, for reasons that aren't entirely understood. It seems to have something to do with a drop in oestrogen levels, such as occurs at the beginning of a menstrual period, though there is no real pattern: migraine can strike before and after periods, or in the middle of the cycle. There are oestrogen receptors in various key areas in the brain involved in pain control. It is likely that this is the basis for menstrual migraine.

Typical pattern of migraine pain

(The darker the shaded area the more intense the pain)

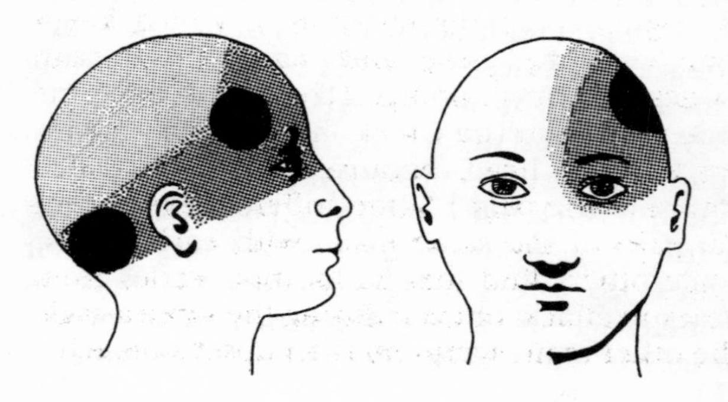

Migraines often improve or disappear during pregnancy and may disappear after menopause (though they may worsen *at* menopause). Hormonal migraines may be treated by administering oestrogen via skin patches (estraderm patches).

Women using oral contraceptives may find their migraines increasing in frequency and severity; others, previously migraine-free, may suddenly start having attacks. However, it doesn't always work this way – some women find themselves free of migraine for the first time in their lives when they start taking the pill. Women who find their migraines either starting, changing in character or dramatically increasing would be advised to discontinue oral contraceptives.

WHAT IS THE PAIN LIKE?

A pain in the head, usually unilateral (one-sided), is the most obvious and worst symptom of migraine – a throbbing ache which keeps time with the pulse and may worsen with movement or straining. (The word migraine is derived from the Greek 'hemicrania', meaning half the head, because of this one-sided nature of the pain.) Some sufferers experience the pain in the same place with each attack, while others find that its location varies from attack to attack, or even during the same attack. The other main symptom is an upset stomach –

nausea and vomiting, after which the sufferer often feels better – which is why migraines are sometimes called sick headaches.

Other migraine symptoms may include visual disturbances (seeing spots, stars, zig-zags and other forms), numbness, tingling and weakness of the limbs, as well as confusion and even an inability to speak properly. Sometimes these symptoms are warning signs (the so-called 'aura'), signals that head pain will soon strike in earnest. The pain may start slowly and build over several hours to a point when most people find it impossible to carry on. Migraineurs typically crave darkness and sleep, wanting nothing more than to lie down in a quiet room until the attack is over. The whole experience may last for many hours or even days.

WHAT CAUSES MIGRAINE?

That's the sixty-four million dollar question. Despite the fact that migraine is one of the most documented complaints in history, we still don't know the answer. We do know that there is a sudden narrowing, then widening, of arteries leading to one side of the head. The stretching of these vessels seems to be the source of the pain, but what makes the arteries contract and dilate in this fashion is unclear.

What makes it even harder to deal with is the fact that the migraine experience – symptoms, triggers and effective treatments – varies widely, according to the individual migraineur. Each case is unique, and must be treated accordingly.

IS THERE A 'MIGRAINE PERSONALITY'?

Many famous people, including Virginia Woolf, John Calvin, Julius Caesar, philosopher Immanuel Kant, Charles Darwin, and Sigmund Freud, have been migraineurs. This has contributed to the popular belief that migraine goes hand-in-hand with brilliance or artistic talent. But migraine is quite unpredictable, striking geniuses and people of average ability alike. However, it is thought that tense, driven and obsessive people may be more susceptible to migraine than others with a happy-go-lucky attitude to life.

TYPES OF MIGRAINE

There are several varieties of migraine, but a high percentage of migraineurs suffer from one of the two major categories: **common migraine** and **classical migraine**.

Common Migraine (Migraine without Aura)

As the name implies, this is the type of migraine suffered by most migraineurs. So-called 'weekend migraines', dietary migraines (see page 25) and menstrual migraines are all examples of common migraine. Premonitory symptoms can include changes in appetite and mood, from euphoria to depression, from hyper-activity to lethargy.

The headache itself is typically throbbing and unilateral, and may be compounded by nausea, vomiting, fever and chills. There may also be a heightening of sensory perceptions (i.e. an exaggerated awareness of light, sound, smell and touch). These symptoms generally develop after the headache starts. Though they may persist for hours and sometimes days, it is rare for the headache to last as long, usually only until the sufferer goes to sleep. She or he may feel weak for some time after the symptoms have subsided.

Classical Migraine (Migraine with Aura)

Classical migraine is the less common main variation of migraine (suffered by about 12 per cent of migraineurs). Attacks tend to be less frequent and briefer than common migraines. The headache starts on one side, as in common migraine, but often spreads to other parts of the head. Accompanying or preceding symptoms include nausea, vomiting and loss of appetite. Pins and needles may be felt down one side of the body and, occasionally, weakness and temporary paralysis. The sufferer may feel confused and have trouble speaking and understanding speech. Such symptoms seldom last for longer than an hour once the headache develops. The most dramatic and distinguishing feature of classical migraine is the visual disturbances often experienced during the aura stage: bright flashing or shimmering lights, wavy lines, concentric circles, blank spots and tunnel vision. These can last for up to an hour, and can be very disturbing, particularly if experienced by children. It's thought that some of the 'visions' described by saints and mystics may have, in fact, been migrainous in origin, such as those recorded in the famous paintings of the visionary nun Hildegard of Bingen (1098–1179), which feature shooting stars and 'fortification spectra' (crenellated) lines similar to the outlines of battlements), often 'seen' during the aura phase.

Other Types of Migraine

- **Basilar Artery Migraine:** Much less common, though similar to classical migraine, this form of migraine mainly affects adolescents. The basilar artery runs along the base of the brain, supplying the brainstem with blood, and it's thought that the migraine is due to a spasm in this artery, depriving some parts of the brain of blood. Basilar artery migraines are characterised by the visual disturbances associated with classical migraine symptoms, as well as giddiness, loss of balance, and slurred speech. The pain strikes mainly in the back of the head.

- **Hemiplegic and Ophthalmoplegic Migraine:** Even rarer variations, in which the pain is relatively mild and, as usual, unilateral. With hemiplegic migraine, as the name suggests, there is a temporary paralysis or weakening of one side of the body. With ophthalmoplegic migraine, there is a temporary paralysis of the eye muscles, resulting in double vision or a drooping eyelid.
- **Retinal Migraine:** Caused when the blood vessels in the retina of one eye go into spasm, resulting in temporary blindness. After vision returns, the victim may experience a lingering, dull ache behind the eye.
- **Abdominal Migraine:** A type of migraine with no headache, only pain in the stomach, sickness and other abdominal disturbances. This type of migraine affects children (see Chapter 9, 'Children's Headaches').

DID YOU KNOW?

Feverfew

There are numerous herbal remedies which are said to heal headache, but the one with the most going for it, at least from the point of view of mainstream medicine, is the weed Feverfew (*Tanacetum parthenium*). Clinical trials seem to indicate some benefits from Feverfew as a migraine treatment; however, it tastes very bitter and can have side effects, including mouth ulcers and a swollen tongue.

WHAT TRIGGERS MIGRAINE?

While the precise causes of migraine are unknown, there are a number of common trigger factors which seem to set off an attack. Many migraineurs are able to identify specific foods, situations or events that bring on headache. These vary enormously – what sets one person's migraine wheel in motion can have no effect on another migraineur – so it's recommended that you keep a migraine diary (see page 85). By jotting down the time, place, and the circumstances surrounding each attack, you will build up a picture of your migraine pattern. Over a period of time, you may well be able to identify the factor – whether it be a particular food, fatigue or stress – that triggers *your* migraine, and work towards avoiding it. This won't cure your migraines or lessen the pain of each attack but, with any luck, you'll suffer far fewer of them. And you will be in control of your headaches, not the other way around. Common migraine triggers include:

- **Food:** Many foods seem to trigger migraine, in particular alcohol, chocolate, cheese and citrus fruits, as well as Monosodium Glutamate (MSG), cured meats (bacon, salami, ham etc.), and fried, fatty foods and spicy foods. None of these items may trigger *your* migraines, but others might, which is why it's worth keeping a diary. Eating *less* can also trigger headaches, particularly in dieters who skip meals. This unwise habit results in low sugar levels, and some migraineurs find they can stop an attack by eating something sweet as soon as they notice the first symptoms.

- **Allergies:** Allergic reactions – to food, animals and other items – and asthma are both known triggers for migraines. If you know what you're allergic to, you can take steps to minimise your exposure; if not, keeping a migraine diary may help you identify it.
- **Change:** Any variation in usual routine can trigger migraine. Many migraineurs suffer 'weekend migraines', which come on at weekends or during holidays, due to the break in workday routine. Times that should be relaxing turn out to be anything but. One way to avoid this trigger is to keep your usual hours as much as possible during your days off – i.e. not staying up or sleeping in later than usual. Try to avoid, wherever possible, extreme highs and lows in your life. By planning a routine that balances work demands with time out for relaxation, exercise and fun, you may be able to avoid those peaks and troughs that can trigger migraine.
- **Physical environment:** Dramatic changes in the weather, working conditions, fumes, smoke and humidity can all trigger migraines. There's not much you can do about the weather, but you can take steps to minimise your exposure to other environmental factors, if only to ask for minor changes to your workplace.

- **Fatigue:** Mental and physical fatigue contribute to tension, which can often be a precipitating factor in migraines as well as tension headaches.
- **Stress:** Emotional upheaval triggers migraines, just as it does tension headaches. It is impossible to go through life without stress, but it is possible to learn to deal with it, to a large extent by making the effort to develop a more relaxed outlook on life. More on this in Chapter 4, 'Learning How to Relax'.
- **Poor health:** Migraine can be associated with recurrent health problems such as anaemia, cystitis, flu, bronchitis and diarrhoea. If you keep coming down with bugs and you've noticed a relationship between feeling poorly and your headaches, don't simply soldier on. Seek medical treatment for the specific complaint and ask for general advice on improving your health – perhaps your diet, exercise regime and other habits need some modification – and your migraines may well improve.

MEDICAL TREATMENT

Migraineurs should seek medical advice for their condition. While it is incurable, there are many medications and other treatments which help minimise attacks or lessen the pain when they occur. Your doctor may refer you to a headache or pain clinic (see page 83, 'Helpful Addresses') which specialises in treating migraines and other headaches and painful conditions in a variety of ways.

As far as medication goes, there are two main approaches to treating migraine. One is to administer painkillers that diminish or 'cover up' the pain, but don't actually stop the attack; that still runs its biological course, as you will discover when the analgesic's effect wears off. There is a wide range of such analgesics, ranging from over-the-counter painkillers to pethidine injections. The second approach is prescribed drugs that act on the immediate causes or triggers of migraines and actually stop the headache. Any migraine medication is more effective the earlier in the attack it is taken – preferably during the aura stage.

There are also drugs which may be taken regularly – not just during the attack – to stop migraines ever developing. Other drugs may be prescribed to treat nausea or other distressing migraine symptoms. Medication may be in the form of tablets to be swallowed, or suppositories.

- **Painkillers:** You can follow the advice given for tension headache – a couple of analgesic tablets containing aspirin or paracetamol, a cup of tea or coffee and a good lie down. Rest is definitely part of the prescription for migraineurs, and many simply have to go to bed, preferably in a quiet, dark room. Some analgesics contain mixtures of aspirin, paracetamol and codeine, caffeine and mild relaxants. This treatment may be effective for some; many others find they need something stronger.

Narcotic analgesics – such as codeine and dihydrocodeine – provide stronger relief, but these can be addictive and can have other unpleasant side effects, such as constipation, nausea and drowsiness, so should be used sparingly and under your doctor's direction. Pethidine, which is given by injection, is a very strong narcotic analgesic, which may be administered at the height of extreme pain.

- **Anti-depressants:** Depression-relieving drugs, such as Tofranil, Trytizol and Prothiaden, may be prescribed, not so much to treat depression as to act on the chemical messengers in the brain which are involved in pain.
- **Non-steroidal Anti-Inflammatory Drugs (NSAIDS):** These work by reducing inflammation and pain, in a similar way to aspirin. Brand names include Nurofen, Naprosyn, Indomethocin and Ponstan.
- **Anti-emetics:** A problem with the stomach upsets that often accompany migraine is that they prevent effective absorption of pain-killing medication. So your doctor may prescribe anti-emetics (anti-sickness drugs) such as Maxolon or Stemetil to solve this problem, as well as treat nausea and vomiting. Some anti-emetics are combined with painkillers.
- **Ergotamine Preparations:** Ergotamine is a very old and effective drug, which works by contracting the migraine-causing dilated blood vessels in the scalp. In effect, it stops

migraines, but will not prevent them recurring. It is, in fact, developed from ergot, a fungus growing on rye plants. Ergot's effects were known in Europe as long ago as the 14th century when it was called St Anthony's Fire, because it was such an effective vasoconstrictor (blood vessel contractor) that a terrible burning sensation, followed by gangrene, could result from eating too much mouldy rye bread! Ergotamine relieves migraine in many patients, but it is addictive and has serious side effects, particularly if used in excess. Because it constricts the veins and arteries, it can cause problems for people with heart disease and vascular problems. Pregnant women should not take it, as it can cause contractions of the uterus and miscarriage. It also *causes* rebound migraines, if abused. It must be used cautiously and under strict medical supervision. Sometimes, ergotamine is mixed with caffeine, anti-histamines and other agents. Brand names include Cafergot, Migral and Ingraine.

- **Preventative Medications:** Some drugs may be prescribed to prevent migraines occurring in the first place. They will not help the pain of an actual attack.

  They must be taken every day, and it may be some time before their beneficial effects are felt. They include:

Beta-blockers These drugs work by relaxing blood vessel walls. They are commonly prescribed to slow the heart rate and lower blood pressure. Beta-blockers like Inderal, Tenormin, Blocadren and Lopresor can all reduce the frequency of migraine attacks. They can have side effects, but must not be discontinued suddenly; they must only be taken under medical supervision.

Calcium channel blockers These drugs work similarly to beta-blockers, expanding the blood vessels by relaxing their walls. Brand names: Plendil, Adalat, Cardene, Dilzem, Tildiem, Motens, Securon, Nimotop, Verapamil. While quite often prescribed, there is some debate among doctors about the usefulness of calcium channel blockers.

Clonidine Another drug, used to treat high blood pressure as well as migraine, which works by relaxing the blood vessel walls, allowing the vessels to dilate. However, once again, there are doubts about its effectiveness as a migraine treatment. Possible side effects include stomach upsets and a dry mouth. Brand names: Catapres and Dixarit.

Methysergide This is probably the most effective prophylactic drug for migraine. It works by constricting the blood vessels and by blocking the action of serotonin, a chemical which signals pain to the brain (including migraine pain). Some migraineurs will become headache-free while taking it; a small percentage cannot tolerate it. It does have side effects, including skin and stomach problems and drowsiness, and must be used only under medical direction. Brand name: Deseril.

Pizotifen This is another drug which works by blocking the action of serotonin. It is effective, widely prescribed and safe, though it can cause hair loss, weight gain (through stimulating the appetite) and drowsiness. Brand name: Sandomigran.

Stop Press – New Drug

Supmatriptan (brand name: Imigran): This drug has been hailed as a major breakthrough in migraine treatment by local neurologists. In trials, it has successfully treated migraine pain in 80 per cent of cases. It works by mimicking the action of serotonin (the chemical messenger which controls pain messages into the brain, among other functions). As we've seen, other migraine medications also work by 'turning off' the brain's pain receptors, but they can affect other body functions affected by serotonin as well, causing disagreeable side effects such as flushing, diarrhoea and stomach upsets. Imigran works on the pain receptors alone, with virtually no side effects.

Self-help for Migraine Sufferers

Many of the same measures that work for tension headaches work for migraines. There seems to be an overlap in the two conditions; migraineurs often suffer from tension headaches, and are sometimes uncertain as to which type they are suffering from at any one point. As with tension headaches, learning the art of relaxation can reduce the frequency and severity of migraine attacks. A variety of relaxation techniques are described in detail in the following chapter. Migraineurs and sufferers of tension headaches should read it carefully, and remember that what works for one may not work for all. Persevere until you have hit on what best helps your headache.

Chapter 4

Learning How to Relax

'I saw a great star most splendid and beautiful, and with it an exceeding multitude of falling stars which the star followed southwards. . . . And suddenly they were all annihilated, being turned into black coals . . . and cast into the abyss.'

– The visionary nun **Hildegard of Bingen** (1098–1180), describing what modern neurologists believe to be visual disturbances typical of classic migraine.

Keeping calm at all times is practically impossible. However, learning to let go is an essential step in preventing headaches developing, and may help to get rid of them, once started.

The stress-busters in Chapter 2 will give quick relief to scrunched-up muscles, but you really need to learn how to relax properly if you are to control your tension, some migraines and other headaches. There's a lot more to relaxing than simply telling yourself to relax, of course. You have to work at it and, like most things in life, the more you practise, the better you get. Relaxation is something of an acquired skill that takes time to master.

You may find it helps to relax in company; if so, you might like to consider a course in meditation, yoga, tai chi, or any other gentle, contemplative exercise. Ask about relaxation courses at your community health centre, nearest large hospital or local health department.

Or you could teach yourself to relax. The following exercises are designed to make you relax deeply, progressively, relaxing every part of the body. It may take a while for you to locate, let alone relax, the various muscles, but don't worry, you'll get the hang of it eventually. Wear comfortable clothing and choose a well-ventilated room with plenty of space for you to stretch out. The important thing is to allow yourself plenty of time – and to perform these exercises regularly, preferably every day.

DEEP RELAXATION

Lie down on the floor or on a very firm bed. Consciously loosen all your muscles, so that your limbs feel like dead weights and your whole body is pushing down heavily on the floor.

Now, keeping the rest of your body relaxed, tighten all the muscles in your feet and legs.

Hold for five counts, then release for five counts. Repeat five times.

- Allow 30 seconds' rest between this and the next and each subsequent step.
- Now repeat the same loosening and tightening exercise for the muscles of your pelvic area and bottom. Repeat five times, remembering to keep the rest of the body relaxed.
- Follow the same procedure for the muscles of your back and torso. Repeat five times.
- Now your arms and hands. Five repeats.
- Now your shoulders and neck. Five repeats.
- Now your facial muscles should be worked individually: relaxing and tightening the muscles of your jaw, your forehead, your scalp and around your eyes in turn. Repeat five times.
- Finally, tense and relax the muscles of your whole body. Repeat five times.

Now let every muscle go, and lie quietly for at least five minutes. Allow your body to go completely limp, feeling that heavy sensation overwhelming your limbs, your body and your head.

As you rest, try to think of something soothing. Imagine you are lying on a beautiful sandy beach, for instance. The warm sun is kissing your body and the leaves in the trees above are rustling in the breeze. Gentle waves lap the shore and all around is safe and tranquil.

Everyone has his or her own escape fantasy – maybe yours is of a stroll in a rainforest, or a swim in a mountain stream. Whatever your fantasy, escape into it completely for five minutes.

Keeping Up the Good Work

Now that you've finished these exercises, you should be feeling calm and refreshed, but it doesn't end there.

For any long-term benefit, it's essential that you practise deep relaxation as often as possible. There is no point in following the routine religiously for a week or two and then giving up because you are feeling better. Relaxation must become an integral and continuous part of your life – and that means all the time, not just when you are doing your exercises.

For instance, try to remember to do regular spot-checks on your posture. How are you standing? Are your back and neck straight, your shoulders and head relaxed?

When you're talking to your boss, are your jaw muscles taut and your stomach in a knot?

Take a deep breath and relax!

You'll find that you can face any situation, however stressful, without knotting up, once you have learned how to relax. Now that you have become aware of warning signs – a tightening of the jaw or scalp; tension in the neck or shoulders – take a few minutes to loosen your muscles. You won't just ward off tension headaches, you'll perform better and finish the day feeling good. Relaxation costs nothing and has no side effects, so there's no excuse not to get cracking. And keep at it!

FACT FILE

Stone-age surgery
Our Neolithic ancestors invented trephining (primitive brain surgery, involving removing circular chunks of skull) to create escape hatches for the evil spirits thought responsible for the pain of headache. Amazingly, many survived this grisly operation, judging by studies of bone regrowth around the resulting holes; but whether their headaches improved is debatable.

OTHER FORMS OF RELAXATION THERAPY

Many forms of pain and stress treatment, including many so-called 'alternative' therapies, are, in fact, versions of relaxation therapy, training the body to let go and/or the mind to turn off. Treatments such as hypnosis, acupuncture and biofeedback seem to work well for some headache sufferers, less well for others. Some orthodox medical practitioners may say that alternative treatments work by the placebo effect (they relieve pain simply because you expect them to), but that doesn't make them any less effective for all that.

Hypnosis

Despite the stereotype of the Svengali hypnotist forcing the subject into actions against his will, this is, in fact, a form of deep relaxation which involves the subject's full co-operation. With the help of a qualified hypnotherapist, the subject is taught to relax until he enters a trance-like state in which he is susceptible to suggestions, but always in control of his own consciousness and actions. Regularly achieving this state takes time and practice, but the benefits are twofold: your muscles automatically relax during a trance, relieving the pain of tension and some other headaches; and it assists you to filter out pain, which is why it is sometimes used to ease the pangs of childbirth or tooth extraction.

Massage

Massage is a wonderful way to relieve muscle tension in the shoulders, neck and head. Professional massages, even facials, are lovely but a bit expensive if indulged in regularly. See if you can talk your partner or friend into giving you one, otherwise you can treat yourself. Use your fingertips or a soft brush to massage the scalp and stimulate the underlying muscles and blood vessels. In both cases, the pattern of stimulation is the same: start at the corners of the eyes and work your way back towards the ears, down the front of the ears, up and over the ears and around to the back of the skull where the large and small neck muscles converge (see diagram).

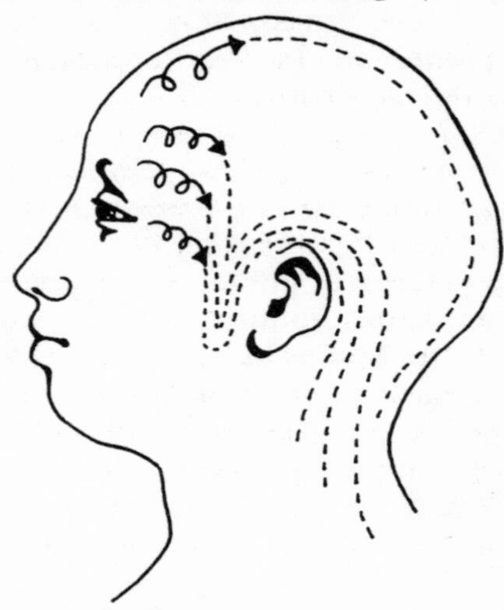

Use fingers or a soft brush to massage the scalp, starting at the corners of the eyes and working backwards around the ears and down to the back of the skull.

Massaging the trapezius muscle in the back (the large ridge of muscle connecting neck and shoulder) also relieves tension, though this can be a bit tricky to do on your own. But if nobody's available to give you a massage, you can use the heel and the fingertips of the right hand to gently rub and manipulate the left shoulder. Repeat with the left hand working the right shoulder.

Acupressure

Acupressure is a self-help treatment that lies somewhere between massage and acupuncture; it involves massaging or manipulating certain 'points' on the head and body, which seems to relieve or head off developing headache pain. The diagrams on the next two pages show the location of these points: use your thumbs or fingertips to deliver a variety of pressures to each. Choose either a steady sustained pressure, a gentle squeeze-and-relax alternation or tiny rotating strokes, whichever feels best for you. This pressure should be applied to each of the points on pages 42 & 43 for 20–30-second periods, to both left and right sides of the head and body. Don't press too hard; just firmly enough to produce a tingling sensation radiating out from each point.

Yoga

An ancient discipline, yoga was developed in India as a complex philosophy as well as an aid to health. It has been adopted in Western countries, primarily for its relaxation techniques. Hatha yoga, exercises involving stretching and slow, graceful movement, as well as breathing exercises, is that most commonly practised in this country. The various yoga positions should be easy to attain without strain, but, because they can be quite complex, seek instruction from a qualified teacher.

ACUPRESSURE POINTS

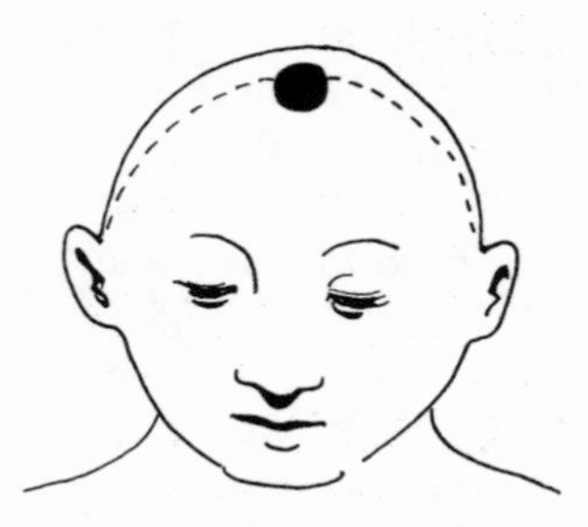

Top of the head: Draw an imaginary line from the tip of your ears to the top of the head. Where that line intersects is the point you're after.

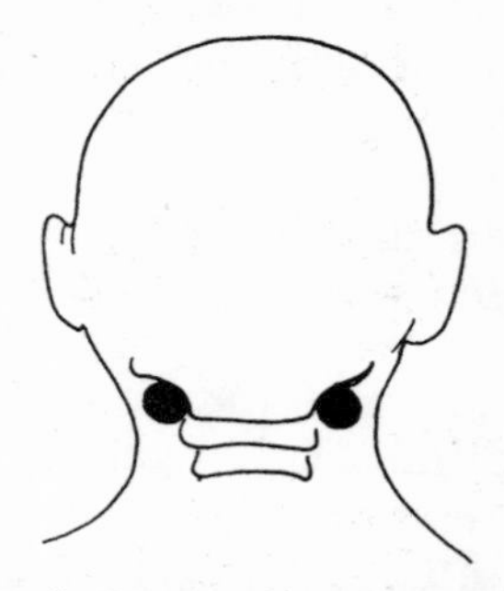

Back of the head: Feel the back of the head level with your earlobes around the hair line for two bumps on either side of the mid-line. Now, move your fingers down about two and a half centimetres under these bumps; apply pressure to these points.

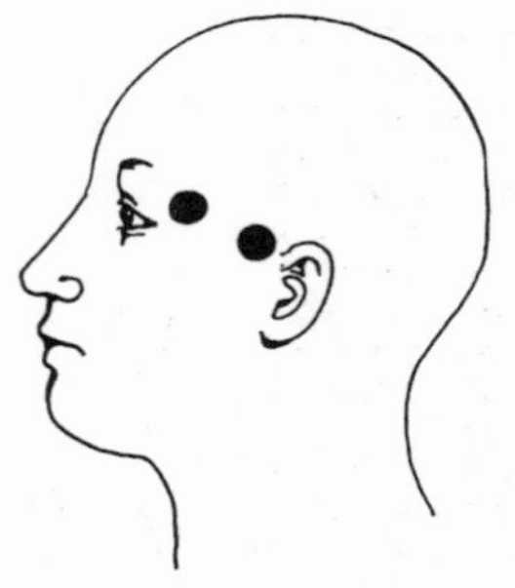

Side of the head: Feel for the slight depression of the skull at each temple behind the eyebrow. Apply gentle, rotating pressure with the tips of your middle fingers.
Front of each ear: Locate the depression in front of the upper earlobes, above the jaw muscle.

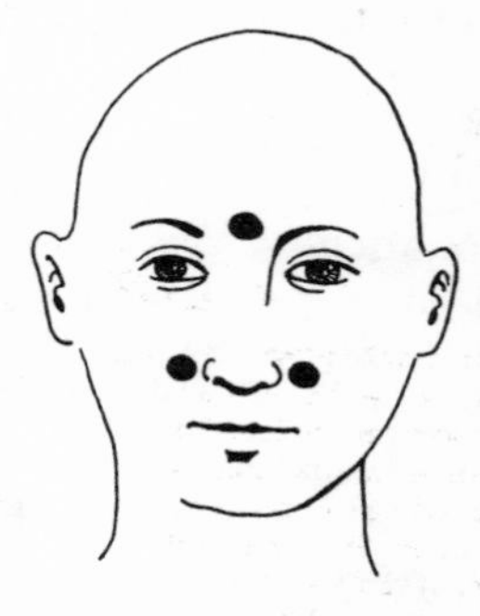

Sinus points: These are found on either side of the nose, slightly above the nostrils and between the eyebrows. Apply gentle pressure on all three points with fingertips.

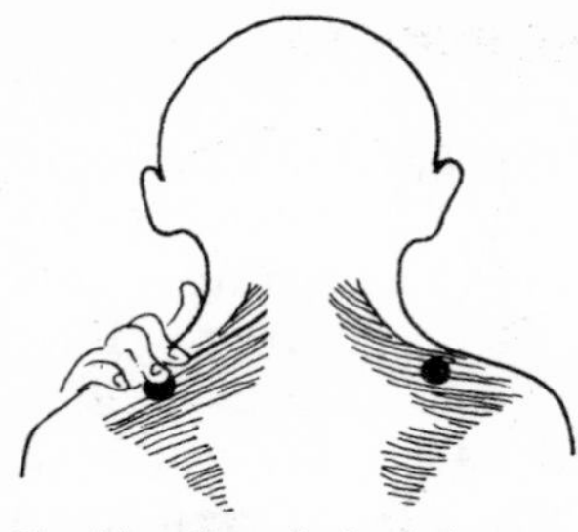

Shoulder: Place the heel of your right hand on the left collarbone, with your thumb resting against your neck, your fingers draped over your shoulder. The tip of your middle finger should now be resting over the point. Apply firm pressure while quickly vibrating or tapping your finger up and down. Repeat with left hand on right shoulder.

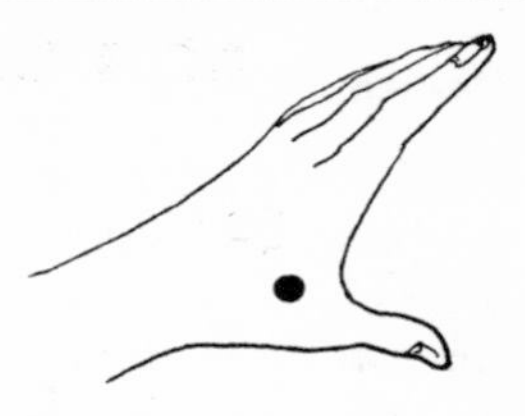

Hand: Stretch the right hand out flat with the thumb extended at a right-angle to the palm. Gently grasp the web of muscle connecting thumb and palm between your left index finger and thumb, with the index finger on the palm side and the thumb on the back of the hand. The tip of the thumb is now on the acupressure point; apply gentle pressure/rotation. Repeat for the other hand.

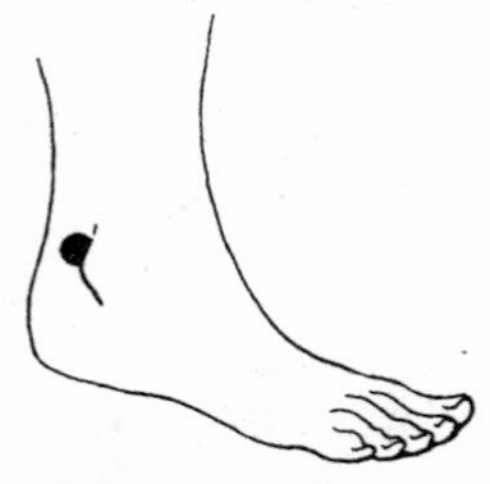

Achilles Tendon: This point is on the outside of the foot just behind the ankle bone, in front of the Achilles Tendon of the heel. Sit down and apply firm pressure, using the middle fingers.

Shin: Place the middle finger of the right hand on the right kneecap and then slide it down to the next lump, which is the head of the shinbone. Now, slide it down the outside of the shinbone about two and a half centimetres, and you will find a spot that is quite sensitive when you press in against the shinbone. Apply pressure and rotation to this point on both legs.

Top of foot: In the depression between the big and second toes, about two and a half centimetres above the web between the toes, firmly massage on both feet.

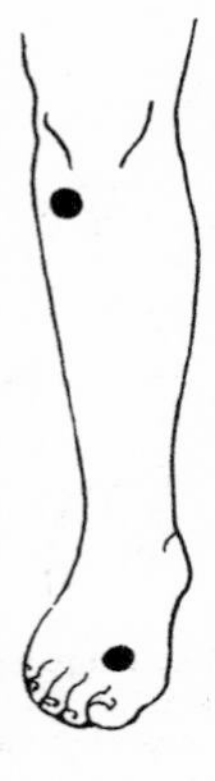

Meditation

There are several types of meditation, most involving concentrating the consciousness on a single focus – it could be a visual image or a repeated word (mantra) – in an attempt to filter out distracting, external stimuli and to attain a more relaxed, detached state of mind. If achieved, this may result in a decreased heart beat and blood pressure and other signs of physical relaxation. Meditation seems to be more effective with sufferers of tension headaches than migraineurs.

DID YOU KNOW?

Acupuncture

This is an ancient Chinese treatment involving piercing points along 'meridians' (imaginary lines drawn across the body's surface said to correspond to life force flow) with slender sterilised needles. Sometimes, a weak electric current is run through the needles. It isn't painful in expert hands and, in fact, has been demonstrated to have an anaesthetic (pain killing) effect for various conditions, including headache. But be sure to check your practitioner out first – it's possible to transmit diseases like Hepatitis B or AIDS through unsterile needles.

Biofeedback

This is a technique using various measuring devices which monitor body functions of which we may normally be unaware, such as changes in muscle tension. By allowing the patient to 'see' these changes, he can learn consciously to control them. Biofeedback can also train patients to modify the brain's alpha rhythms, helping to promote relaxation. This technique is used to help control migraine pain, among other things, and to reduce the need for medication.

Exercise

One of the best and easiest ways to relax is to increase your exercise level. A brisk walk or quick swim is a great tension-reliever, as well as benefiting your health in many other ways. Make sure the exercise is sustained and moderate – an overambitious exercise plan can actually cause headaches (see Chapter 8, 'Other Headaches').

Chapter 5
Cluster Headaches

> *'When the head aches, all the body is out of tune.'*
>
> – From **Don Quixote** by Miguel de Cervantes Saavedra (1547–1616)

Cluster headaches, like migraines, are 'vascular' headaches, in that they are associated with changes in the blood vessels. The term 'cluster' refers to the odd way these headaches strike – they occur in regular bouts, or clusters, each lasting for days, weeks or months.

WHO GETS THEM?

Cluster headaches are relatively rare – affecting less than one in a thousand Britons – and probably get more attention than they warrant, because of the dramatic and often frightening form the pain takes. Unlike migraine and tension headaches, men are the main sufferers – about 85 per cent of cluster-headache victims are male. Attacks frequently commence in puberty but can develop anytime between 10 and 30 years of age. It's thought that Thomas Jefferson, author of the Declaration of Independence, suffered from cluster headaches; certainly, every victim of this type of headache (and others) will empathise with his doleful words: 'An attack of the "periodical" headache came upon me about a week ago, rendering me as yet unable to write or read without great pain.'

Typical pattern of cluster-headache pain

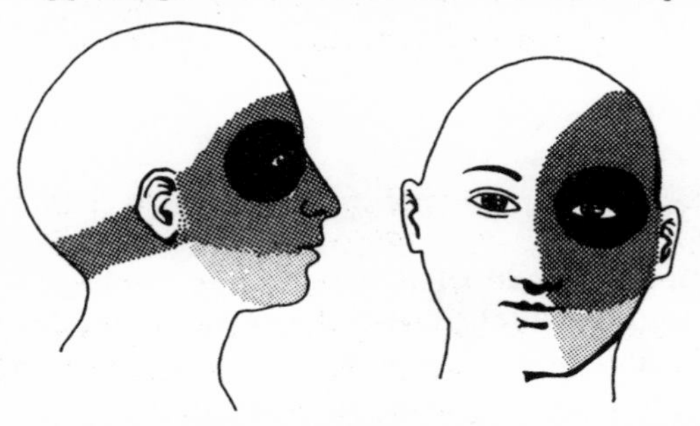

(The darker the shaded area the more intense the pain)

WHAT IS THE PAIN LIKE?

The pain of cluster headaches can be quite excruciating, centring around one eye and often radiating downwards over the same side of the face or upwards to the forehead and temple. The pain is often described as 'piercing' or 'tearing' and is intense and continuous, not throbbing. It has been known to make its victims run around, clutching their heads. They don't want to lie in darkened rooms like migraineurs, but have to move or pace about. The pain strikes suddenly and in rapid succession; the victim may experience several headaches daily for weeks, each lasting anywhere from 10 minutes to a couple of hours. The headaches then disappear as quickly as they came, only to strike again months or years later in the same pattern as before. These bouts are so regular that some victims say they can set their watches by them, and even find themselves being woken by the pain at the same time every night.

Other Symptoms

The affected side of the face and eyelids may swell and the eyelids may droop. The eye, itself, often reddens and waters, and the nose may run. The neck may also become painful. Nausea or vomiting rarely feature in cluster headaches, unlike migraines. However, they are sometimes mistaken for migraines, or for attacks of tic douloureux (see Chapter 6).

WHAT CAUSES CLUSTER HEADACHES?

The cause is unknown, but, because they strike in such regular cycles – victims can, say, be hit at 4am every morning in May – the body-clock mechanism is probably implicated. (This is one of the primitive functions controlled by the hypothalamus, the part of the brain which regulates the autonomic nervous system.) The eye symptoms and others suggest that certain nerves in the head may be involved, but nobody really knows.

MEDICAL TREATMENT

Medication for cluster headaches is similar to that prescribed for migraines. It should only ever be taken under medical supervision.

- **Methysergide (Deseril):** This benefits about 7 out of every 10 sufferers of cluster headaches, but to be effective must be taken in larger doses than those given to migraineurs. Because it will generally be taken for relatively short periods, there is less concern about side effects for cluster-headache victims than migraineurs.
- **Ergotamine preparations:** These aren't quite as effective as for migraines, because the duration of each headache is shorter and there is less time for the ergotamine to take effect. However, it can be used as a preventative; once the bouts have been monitored, ergotamine may be taken prior to the next expected episode. Ergotamine seems to become less effective with each subsequent bout of cluster headache.
- Corticosteroids (steroidal drugs which reduce inflammation, such as Prednisone): These effectively arrest a bout, but should not be taken for more than a couple of weeks so as to

avoid the risk of quite severe side effects. The usual procedure is to start with large doses, and then taper them off over the next few days.

- **Oxygen:** Inhaling 100 per cent oxygen is very effective at getting rid of the pain of cluster headaches. Frequent sufferers could benefit from installing oxygen apparatus – a cylinder, valve and a mask – at home or at work to deal with attacks.

Self-help for Cluster Headaches

Alcohol seems to be a very definite trigger for cluster headaches, as it is for migraines. Victims should abstain from alcohol for the entire cluster-headache period, and should generally be wary about drinking. Seek the advice of your doctor about your alcohol intake. Cluster headaches seem to strike men who smoke, in particular, another reason to give up.

Chapter 6

Tic Douloureux (Trigeminal Neuralgia)

Tic douloureux is French for 'woeful spasm', and it certainly causes its victims considerable woe. It is an intense jab of pain, not unlike that of cluster headaches, which affects parts of the face suddenly, briefly – and excruciatingly.

WHO GETS IT?

Once again, this is a type of headache suffered mostly by women, for reasons not understood. Female victims outnumber males by two to one. Sufferers are typically middle-aged; tic douloureux is rarely seen in anyone under the age of 40.

WHAT DOES THE PAIN FEEL LIKE?

It strikes in sudden, excruciating stabs, to one side of the gum, cheek, chin or forehead. Attacks are brief, usually lasting seconds, but may recur in repeated attacks over weeks, disrupting sleep and driving sufferers to distraction, some even to suicide.

WHAT CAUSES TIC DOULOUREUX?

This painful spasm is caused by a change of the impulse patterns in the trigeminal nerve, a major nerve running from brain stem to the front of the head and face (see illustration). It has three major branches, hence the name. Sometimes, impulses to this nerve misfire, sending off an uncontrolled barrage of impulses and causing intense, lightning-like bolts of pain, as brief as they are agonising. Why these abnormal impulses occur is not really understood, but they can be triggered by cold or wind on the face, pressure on the face, as well as by such ordinary movements as chewing, talking, shaving, blowing the nose, laughing or brushing the teeth. Some people are so sensitive that they give up washing the affected part of the face.

Typical pattern of tic douloureux pain

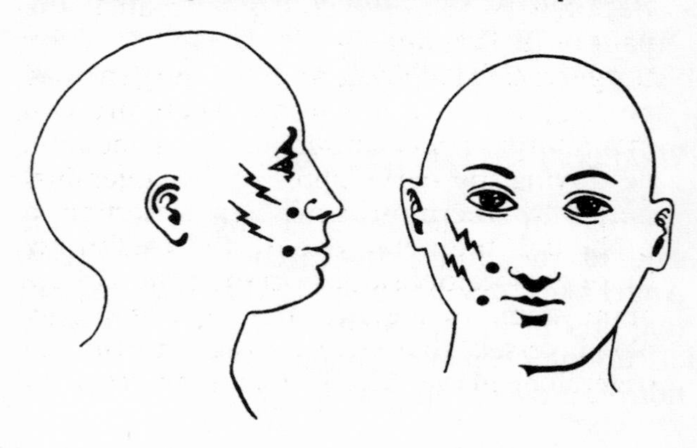

Dental problems may also be a factor, with infection or inflammation causing pressure on the trigeminal nerve. It's thought that the hardening of the arteries, which accompanies ageing, may also play a part.

TREATMENT

- **Check your teeth:** It's worth having a dental examination to make sure that the pain is not being caused by a mal-alignment of your jaw.
- **Avoid trigger factors** such as cold or wind, as much as possible.
- **Medication:** Because of certain similarities to the spasms of epilepsy, anti-epileptic drugs like Tegretol have been successful in treating tic douloureux. However, their effectiveness seems to decline with regular use, and they can have side effects, like weight gain, drowsiness and nausea. The anti-spastic drug Baclofen is also prescribed to reduce the pain of tic douloureux.
- **Surgery:** If drugs bring no relief, surgery may be suggested as a last resort. There are two main surgical procedures for this condition: destroying the nerve fibres of the trigeminal nerve by thermo-coagulation (inserting a probe into the nerve ending and cauterising it); or exploratory surgery in the region of the brain stem, to identify and reposition any blood vessels that may be pressing on the trigeminal nerve. The former may result in

facial numbing and a damaged blink reflex; but the latter is a major, serious surgical procedure.

The three major branches of the trigeminal nerve

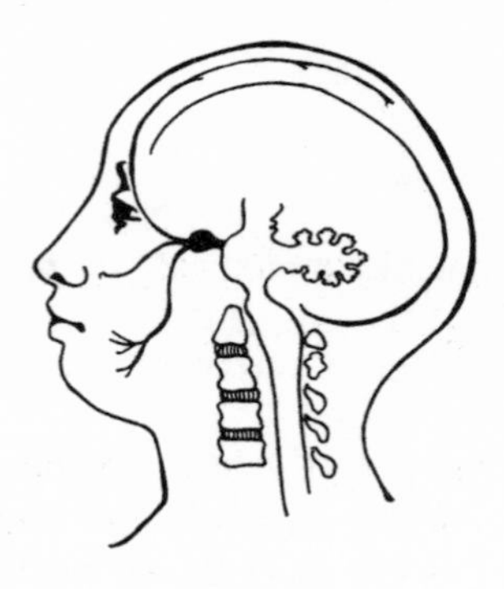

OTHER TYPES OF NEURALGIA

A similar type of pain can result from shingles. This is a painful disease caused by the herpes zoster virus, which infects the nerve roots, resulting in welts of painful, itching blisters around the body along the nerve paths. If the trigeminal nerve is involved, pain similar to that of tic douloureux can result. Surgery doesn't work with post-herpetic neuralgia, as the neuralgia caused by shingles is called. Treatment is difficult after the event, though corticosteroids like Prednisone administered during the active phase of shingles, before neuralgia has set in, may help prevent it.

Chapter 7

Sinus Headaches

'A crown is no cure for the headache.'
– Old English saying

The sinuses are the large, bony cavities in the skull behind the nose, cheeks and eyebrows. Their presence is what gives resonance to the voice – they act as a virtual sound box. The sinuses are particularly sensitive to dust, wind, pollen, cigarette smoke and air-conditioning and central heating. They are normally full of air but, sometimes, as a result of infection such as the common cold or from diseased upper teeth, their mucous membranes become swollen and inflamed, resulting in an uncomfortable pain in the face and head.

WHAT DOES THE PAIN FEEL LIKE?

The sinuses fill with fluid, causing a dull pain over the forehead, cheeks and upper jaw bone. These areas may be tender to the touch. The pain is often worst first thing in the morning, improving as the day wears on. It usually increases on bending, coughing or with changes in pressure, such as experienced during flying or diving. This condition is called sinusitis. It is usually a temporary ailment, clearing up within a few weeks, but can become chronic.

Typical pattern of sinus-headache pain

(The darker the shaded area the more intense the pain)

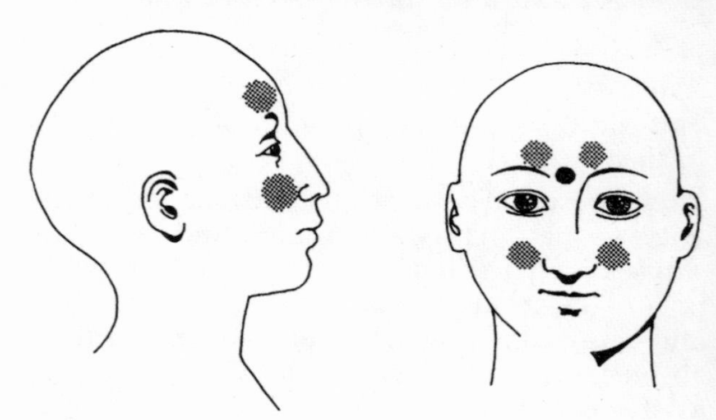

MEDICAL TREATMENT

If sinusitis is severe or lasts longer than a day or so, you should consult your doctor, who may examine you to see whether the infection is resulting from teeth problems, and may order X-rays to see if the sinuses are blocked (they will show up as cloudy patches on the X-ray film if they are). You may be prescribed antibiotics for any infection.

Further Treatment

If the sinusitis does not respond to antibiotics, or has become chronic, you may be referred to an ear, nose and throat surgeon for an operation to open the sinuses. This involves making a hole between sinus and the mouth or nose, allowing it to drain. However, sinusitis does tend to be a recurrent condition.

Self-help for Sinus Headaches

There is some debate over whether the headache suffered by people with sinus problems actually relates to the sinus, or is a form of tension headache. Either way, it can't hurt to treat the infected sinuses.

- **Steam:** The old-fashioned remedy of steam inhalation should help loosen the mucous and relieve the congestion causing the pain. You can simply pour boiling water into a deep bowl or basin, and lean over it, with your head draped in a towel to hold in the steam, or you could rent or buy a commercial vaporiser, available from many pharmacies. Eucalyptus or menthol added to the water enhances the decongestant effect. Steam inhalation is particularly effective if followed up with dry heat – i.e. sitting in front of a radiator or an infrared lamp. Hot compresses on forehead or cheeks help soothe sinus pain.
- **Decongestants:** Nasal decongestants, purchased over the counter from pharmacies,

will also afford temporary relief from sinus headache. They should be taken while lying down with the head tilted back to allow the drops to run to the back of the nose. Once the nostril is clear, sit up and gently blow your nose (if you blast away when both nostrils are blocked, you risk forcing the infection up into your middle ear). Clear one nostril at a time. Constant sniffing, irritating as it may seem, is actually quite a good way to clear sinuses. Remember that decongestants should be used judiciously, as overuse can result in 'rebound' congestion and an even more severe headache.

- **Drink plenty of fluids:** Hot drinks help loosen mucus; soup or tea, those old stand-bys for colds, are ideal.
- **Medication:** Aspirin can help relieve the pain and reduce any accompanying fever.
- **Acupressure:** This may assist sinus headaches as well as migraines and tension headaches. By applying pressure on the points for sinus (as well as the other headache points – as described on pages 42–43), you may achieve a temporary, but noticeable, reduction in pain.

Prevention

- Minimise your exposure to dust and other irritants.
- If you're a smoker, quit now. Tobacco smoke irritates the lining of the nasal and sinus cavities.

Chapter 8

Other Headaches

You may feel the pain of some headaches in your head, but they don't always start there. A multitude of health problems can cause headache, including:

BLOOD PRESSURE

Sudden rises in blood pressure, such as can occur during exercise, may cause headache. The pain will typically be severe throbbing, and strike on both sides of the back or front of the head.

People with hypertension (high blood pressure) sometimes wake with headaches, which wear off after they get up and get cracking. Not everyone with high blood pressure gets headaches, nor does everyone with headaches have high blood pressure; however, hypertensive people seem more susceptible to migraines and, as we've seen, medication to control blood pressure may help control headaches for some people.

EYE STRAIN

People hit with headache often wonder if something is wrong with their eyes. Eye strain can be a cause of headache, particularly if it is caused by an imbalance of the eye muscles. This can cause a constant struggle to focus, particularly when reading, writing, watching television or driving. You may see double when you're tired and unable to control your focus. All this effort can bring on a headache centred around the eyes. If you're having this problem, the obvious course is a visit to an ophthalmologist or optician, who may prescribe eye exercises to tone the muscles.

Pain in the eyes of a more severe and serious kind may be caused by glaucoma, resulting from increased pressure of fluid within the eyeball. The pain, usually very severe, may be mistaken for migraine because it is centred in the eye and can radiate over the forehead. If suffering eye pain, you should promptly consult an ophthalmologist, who will be able to detect glaucoma by measuring the pressure within the eyeball. Immediate attention is essential; if glaucoma is neglected, blindness can result. Treatment, involving drugs or surgery to drain the eye, is usually successful. Glaucoma normally strikes people middle-aged or older; it's a good idea to have your eyes regularly checked from the age of 50 onwards.

DENTAL PROBLEMS

- **Infection:** The pain of an infected tooth may be referred to the trigeminal nerve, causing pain in upper and lower jaw and gums. Your dentist will probably X-ray the painful area to determine if infection is causing the trouble.
- **The bite:** Pain in the temple or ear can be caused by an imbalance of the bite, due to missing teeth or an overlapping of the teeth on one side, which puts pressure on the other jaw. The pain caused by this constant strain can radiate up to the temples, and the area in front of the ear becomes painful to the touch. If you suspect your bite is unbalanced, consult your dentist. He or she will arrange appropriate treatment to correct it.
- **Jaw clenching:** Tense people tend to clench their jaws, which also puts strain on the joints of the jaw. You may notice, after a stressful interview or a row with your partner, that your jaw muscles are aching, with the pain spreading to the front of the ear and up to the top of the head. Obviously, you should check out any sort of jaw or tooth problem with your dentist but, if it seems that your problems are due to or increased by tension, it may be wise to try relaxation therapy. Follow the exercises outlined in Chapter 4, or perhaps, after discussion with your GP, he or she may feel it appropriate to refer you to a psychologist or psychiatrist to get right to the root of the problems causing your tension.

ARTHRITIS

Arthritis in the neck, such as commonly occurs in older people, can cause the muscles to go into spasm, resulting in headache. The pain may spread from the back of the head to the eyes or temples. There is no cure for this problem, but the pain may be treated with muscle-relaxant medication, head massage or wearing a surgical collar.

LOW BLOOD SUGAR

People suffering from diabetes or carbohydrate intolerance may have low blood sugar levels from time to time. This can result in a slowing down of sugar supplies to the brain, which is fuelled by glucose, a sugar. It doesn't take kindly to the deprivation, and migraines may result. Stringent dieting can have the same effect, so try not to skip meals.

ICE-CREAM HEADACHES

It's unfair, isn't it? Eating ice-cream doesn't just make you fat, it can make your head hurt. Some people, particularly those susceptible to migraine, find that eating ice-cream causes headache, usually at the front of the head, but sometimes in the temple or over the ear or at the usual site of migraine pain. It's thought that the sensation of intense cold from the ice-cream causes referred pain via the trigeminal nerve endings. You can also get an ice-cream headache from eating other very cold foods, or from immersing the head in cold water. The solution: abstain from eating cold foods, obviously – or, at least, swallow them quickly, without holding them in the mouth, where they're closer to the nerve endings.

DID YOU KNOW?

Oldie but goodie!
Aspirin is the first line of defence against many types of headache, and is much stronger medicine than many people realise. It's one of a family of drugs, called the salicylates, which have been in use since the Stone Age. Salicylates are naturally present in many trees and shrubs, as the Romans realised when they made painkilling potions out of boiled willow bark. The ancient Greek physician Hippocrates (after whom the Hippocratic oath is named) recommended willow derivatives to relieve pain, fever and the pangs of childbirth, and the Red Indians used them to treat headache, fever and lumbago. Today, aspirin is the most widely used drug in the world.

EXERCISE HEADACHES

Inactive people who start a vigorous exercise programme may find their efforts rewarded, not by increased fitness, but by a throbbing headache and feelings of nausea. During exertion, the muscles require more blood, causing an expansion of the blood vessels (vasodilation), as experienced in migraine. If your fitness routine is causing you headaches, take it as a sign to slow down; as your strength improves, your headaches should wane. It is always advisable to take any new exercise regime slowly, building up your resilience over time.

Migraine sufferers can find that participating in physically and mentally competitive sport triggers attacks. If so, it may be time to find less strenuous and demanding pastimes.

If you get a headache after other physical exertion, such as lifting a heavy weight or bending down, this may be caused by problems in the cervical spine or high blood pressure and you should seek medical advice.

SEX HEADACHES

'Not tonight, dear, I have a headache . . .' There can be a lot of truth in that hoary old chestnut, although the headache is likely to strike <u>during</u> sex, not beforehand as an excuse to put it off. That's right, intercourse can cause headaches (among other things). Over 2,500 years ago, Hippocrates wrote of the pain caused by 'immoderate venery' (sexual indulgence), but you don't have to have been overdoing it to be struck by a terrible stabbing or throbbing pain in the head around orgasm. Sufferers sometimes think they're having a stroke. This has occurred, though rarely, and, because of the slight possibility of underlying vascular disorders, you should probably stop what you're doing and get yourself medically checked out.

However, this embarrassing phenomenon is much more likely to be due to a sudden increase in blood pressure at the climax of sexual activity (during orgasm, blood pressure can climb by as much as 80 per cent and the heart beat can triple its rate). The pain can last from a matter of minutes to days; it may increase slowly with sexual excitement, or arrive like a thunderclap at the point of orgasm.

It's thought that sex headaches can also be triggered by emotional factors, such as fear of pregnancy, disease or guilt.

Whether physical or emotional in origin, people afflicted with sex headaches should discuss the problem with their doctor. If the cause is emotional, you may be referred to a psychologist to help you sort out your feelings about sex. If it is a physical reaction to orgasm, there are medical preparations that may help. Ergotamine tartrate or Indocid may head off headache, if taken before sex; however, because this type of headache is so unpredictable – it can strike at any age and may cease as suddenly as it started – that prevention is difficult. Your only real consolation is the knowledge that sex headaches are pretty uncommon.

HANGOVER HEADACHES

Have you ever woken up feeling shaky and nauseous, head thumping and throat dry? Does your mouth feel like the bottom of a birdcage? It sounds like you had one or two glasses too many the night before, because you have the classic symptoms of a hangover.

What causes hangovers? Alcohol causes blood vessels to dilate, which combines with other factors, such as disturbances in blood sugar levels, to cause headache and other symptoms. It's not just the alcohol, but the congeners mixed with it – chemicals that add different flavours, aromas and colours to different drinks – that you need to be wary of. Certain substances are quite toxic and probably contribute more to the hangover than the booze itself. Other elements associated with heavy drinking don't help, either – noisy, smoke-filled pubs, lack of sleep, loud music, the excitement of a big night out all contribute to headache.

How to avoid hangover headache? There's one simple solution – stop drinking! If you must drink, at least do it carefully. Try to drink in a relaxed atmosphere and make sure that you have food in your stomach. It's a good idea to drink a large glass of milk before going to a party and, when you arrive, think moderation.

If all these careful preparations haven't worked and you've woken up with a humdinger, analgesics and antacid tablets will help reduce headache, stomach acidity, nausea and heartburn – particularly if you follow them up with a cup of tea or coffee, some rest and a solid meal.

DID YOU KNOW?

Crockery crocodile
Migraine is mentioned in the oldest known medical manuscript, the Ebers papyrus, discovered at Thebes, Egypt, last century. It describes it as 'a sickness of half the head'. The ancient Egyptians treated migraine by tying a ceramic crocodile, with herbs stuffed into its mouth, to the head of the patient. The compression of the temples, caused by the tie, was undoubtedly more effective in getting rid of the pain than the crocodile.

REBOUND HEADACHES

If you frequently take substances that cause the blood vessels to contract – caffeine-containing drinks like coffee, some analgesics and other medications, such as ergotamine preparations – this can cause a rebound effect. The vessels 'snap back' by expanding, causing headache instead of curing it. Sudden withdrawal from such substances has the same effect, which is why heavy coffee drinkers trying to quit often get headaches. Seek your doctor's advice, but your wisest course is probably to taper off whatever is causing the rebound headache, not stop cold turkey.

HEAD INJURIES

Head injuries are very common, ranging in severity from minor bumps to serious damage sustained in a car accident. Headache often follows concussion or whiplash injuries, and there's a whole class of headaches called 'footballer's headache', resulting from blows received while playing sport. Such headaches tend to be migrainous, possibly because the injuries affect the action of blood vessels in the head. Migraineurs seem more susceptible to headache after head injury, perhaps for this reason.

Lasting headache is quite common following head injuries, but paradoxical as it may sound, it probably results from emotional causes – distress or trauma from the accident, for example – rather than from physical ones. This doesn't mean the pain isn't real, just that the treatment will be different than if the cause was an ongoing physical problem.

However, headache following injury requires immediate medical attention if it worsens rapidly or the victim seems sleepy – symptoms which point to a blood clot putting pressure on the brain.

Chapter 9

Children's Headaches

'Mummy, my head hurts' . . . 'I feel funny' . . . these are cries with which any parent is all too familiar. And they dread them; the dementing thing about children's headaches is that little children often can't describe them properly, if at all, leaving the parent prey to all sorts of horrible imaginings.

- **Infections:** Headaches are common in young children – particularly between the ages of 4 and 10 – but very rarely serious. In most cases, they are a symptom of common infectious childhood diseases, such as mumps, measles or chickenpox, or illnesses such as influenza, gastroenteritis, even simple colds. Such headaches are usually experienced in the front of the head and develop very quickly. The child is often irritable, uninterested in food, feverish and running a high temperature.
- **Treatment in the home:** The headache is often the first symptom to appear, making diagnosis difficult in the absence of spots or other

obvious signs of illness. Your best bet is to take the child's temperature to see if it is raised, and pack him off to bed. If he is feverish, encourage him to drink lots of fluids. You could also give him paracetamol to relieve the pain and help reduce the temperature. Never give aspirin to a child under the age of 12. The headache will probably diminish over an hour or so, though other symptoms may appear – such as spots, coughs, sniffles, vomiting or diarrhoea.

DID YOU KNOW?

Wisdom born of pain

Even the gods are not immune to headache, according to the Greek myths. Jupiter, father of all the gods, was struck down with an appalling headache. The pain was so bad that he begged Vulcan, the god of blacksmiths, to split his skull open with an axe. Vulcan kindly obliged, and out stepped Minerva, the goddess of wisdom – wisdom born of pain. This myth underlines the common belief that headaches are somehow related to high intelligence. This is an idea that's been given credence by many writers about headache (who are often headache victims themselves), but there isn't any real foundation for it.

- **When to call the doctor:** If you are even mildly concerned, you should consult your doctor, if only to relieve your own mind. If a childhood infection is diagnosed, a course of antibiotics with aspirin or paracetamol may be prescribed. You should certainly seek medical advice if the child's headache persists, is very severe or won't respond to painkillers.

TENSION HEADACHES

These are uncommon in young children, though they should be investigated if they occur, as they may be symptomatic of social problems such as family troubles or bullying at school. If you're certain the problem doesn't lie within the home, then perhaps you should approach your child's teacher to find out if all is well at school. It's always possible, however, if a child is unhappy at school, that he is using the excuse of a headache to wangle days off. Make sure you're not being manipulated!

Older children swotting for major exams are more susceptible. They should be encouraged to take plenty of rest and work out a sensible long-term study plan, not wait until the last moment, then attempt absurd all-night cramming sessions before the big day.

MIGRAINE

Children suffer migraine more often than is realised. Watch out for such symptoms as recurring headaches, particularly at times of high excitement, and especially if linked with nausea, vomiting and lack of appetite. As with adults' migraines, children's migraines are usually unilateral, either to the side of the head or over one eye. The visual side effects that occur in classical migraine are seldom experienced by children, although, if they do develop, they can be extremely frightening for the child, requiring lots of reassurance and comfort. Try to get the child to tell you what he's seeing as precisely as possible at the time; this will assist your doctor, as the child may well have forgotten by the time you've got him to the surgery.

About 20 per cent of migrainous children suffer from abdominal pain. Such pain, and vomiting, may be the only symptoms of a migraine attack, and there may be no headache at all. A number of children who suffer abdominal migraine will go on to develop either common or classical migraine as adults.

Although in adult life four times as many women suffer from migraines as men, during childhood boys are equally as vulnerable as girls. The big switch comes at puberty, when the female hormones implicated in migraine become more active. However, the migraines are quite likely to cease altogether somewhere around 10–12.

Treatment

Simple analgesics are usually very effective with children's migraines, as are small doses of non-steroidal anti-inflammatory drugs (NSAIDS) like Naprosyn. Your doctor may recommend anti-sickness medication for the nausea, but may be reluctant to prescribe other migraine medication for a child. It's recommended that parents react to migraine attacks as calmly as possible, so as not to increase the child's anxiety.

WARNING – CHILDREN AND MEDICINE DON'T ALWAYS MIX!

If you regularly suffer from headaches, you may have assembled quite a medicine chest for yourself. Many headache preparations are extremely effective, but are quite potent drugs, which must be consumed with caution – even plain old aspirin. Many of these drugs are not suitable for children. Of those that are, children's dosages may vary markedly from adults' dosages. Seek your doctor's or pharmacist's advice before administering any medication to children, and be sure to follow your doctor's instructions and/or the directions on the packet before taking any headache preparation yourself. It goes without saying that all medications, even the most innocuous-seeming over-the-counter painkiller, should be kept out of the reach of children.

WHEN TO WORRY

Although rare, headache may signal a number of serious diseases in children, such as encephalitis, meningitis, tumour, cysts and abscesses. Seek medical advice immediately if your child gets a headache out of the blue and then develops further symptoms, such as a drooping eyelid, fever, persistent vomiting, stiffness of the neck, paralysis, delirium, difficulties with breathing, coma, confusion or seeing double.

Also seek advice if the headache is associated with fits or fainting, or follows a head injury. You should also be concerned if the child is waking with headaches, or the headaches are progressively worsening. Serious causes of headache and the treatments are covered in more detail in the following chapter.

Chapter 10

When to Hit the Panic Button

There is an almost universal human tendency to over-react to painful symptoms, and many of us imagine the worst when headache strikes. The most frequent fears are that the headache signals a brain tumour or a stroke. While headache can be a symptom of some very nasty problems indeed, these are quite rare; the overwhelming majority of headaches, as we've seen, have relatively 'innocent' causes, such as tension. However, it's as well to be familiar with symptoms of serious disorders, if only to put your mind at rest about your headache.

And remember, if you're in any way concerned about headaches, either with yourself or your children, you should seek medical advice, regardless of whether you think it's serious or not. In general, it's wise to consult your doctor about <u>any</u> headache which lasts longer than 24 hours and/or doesn't respond to painkillers or prescribed medication.

BRAIN TUMOUR

A brain tumour is a mass growing in the brain, which may be benign or malignant (cancerous). Treatment usually involves surgery, radiotherapy or chemotherapy to remove or shrink the tumour.

Headaches are a symptom of brain tumour, but not all tumour victims will experience them. A tumour won't cause headache until it has grown large enough to put pressure on arteries in the brain. In some areas of the brain, a tumour can grow quite large before causing such pressure, if any, but headache strikes sooner or later with most tumours. The pain usually strikes in the same place, is worse in the morning, is not exceptionally severe (often not as painful as a bad migraine), and may increase with straining (coughing or sneezing).

It's particularly suspicious if such headaches strike someone normally headache-free, if the pain is increasing steadily, or if the usual pattern of headache changes. Other worrying symptoms include signs of neurological damage, such as:

- **Drowsiness**
- **Blurred or double vision**
- **Weakness or numbness of limbs**
- **Loss of balance**
- **Slurred speech**
- **Epileptic fits accompanied by headache**

- **Sudden or gradual change of personality or behaviour**
- **Persistent vomiting, especially in the mornings**

You should see your doctor immediately you notice any of these symptoms. He or she may order a CAT scan – a form of X-ray of the brain – to check for a tumour.

All that being said, it is important to remember that very, very few people with headaches turn out to have brain tumours.

STROKE

Strokes are caused by a blockage (thrombosis) or haemorrhage of a blood vessel in the brain, interrupting the blood supply to the brain and damaging it. This damage depends on which part of the brain the stroke occurs in: if in the left side of the brain, speech will probably be impaired; paralysis may occur, affecting the opposite side of the body to the affected part of the brain. Stroke doesn't usually strike before middle age. It is generally a result of untreated high blood pressure, though heredity and arteriosclerosis (hardening of the arteries) also play a part.

Many stroke victims suffer no headache at all, though about one in three will experience a headache just beforehand. If the stroke is caused by a haemorrhage, pain and stiffness may be felt in the neck and head. If caused by a clot blocking the artery, the victim may experience headache in the back or side of the head. Other warning signals to watch out for include:

- **Pins and needles down one side of the body**
- **Paralysis or weakness of one side of the face or body**
- **Dizziness**
- **Blurred vision**
- **Loss of balance**
- **Confusion or drowsiness**

Seek medical help immediately you notice such symptoms.

The symptoms of migraine are sometimes confused with stroke. Migraine victims who find their symptoms increased by the contraceptive pill may be advised to find another form of contraception, as there is an increased risk of stroke associated with the pill.

ANEURYSMS

Aneurysms are small swellings or balloonings of the artery walls. They may be caused by congenital weakness, disease or hardening of the arteries. High blood pressure places extra strain on aneurysms, and they may enlarge and rupture. The blood vessel most often affected is the aorta (the large artery leading from the left ventricle of the heart), but aneurysms may also affect blood vessels in the brain. If an aneurysm on a cerebral artery bursts, causing bleeding into the brain, it will produce a type of stroke. Plenty of people have aneurysms without being aware of it or experiencing any symptoms; however, anyone with a known aneurysm should be medically monitored, particularly as they age, as the consequences if it ruptures are potentially very serious. Aneurysms can be corrected by surgery.

TEMPORAL ARTERITIS

This is a low-grade inflammation of blood vessels in the scalp, causing reddening and tenderness around those vessels, or a dull ache on the sides of the head. This may be accom-

DID YOU KNOW?

Through a Looking Glass Darkly
The Victorian author Lewis Carroll (real name Charles Dodgson) was a martyr to migraine of a rare variety, symptoms of which include distorted or changing perception of shape and size. It's thought his experiences may have partly inspired his most famous books, *Alice's Adventures in Wonderland* and *Through The Looking Glass*, particularly the 'drink me – eat me' passages, where Alice feels herself growing or shrinking uncontrollably. His migraines, however, seem to have developed later in life.

panied by general aches and pains and other flu-like symptoms. The jaw muscles may ache while chewing. The condition, which is relatively rare, usually affects middle-aged or older people. It is treated with steroids (anti-inflammatory drugs). Prompt medical attention is essential, as untreated arteritis can progress to the ophthalmic artery (which supplies blood to the retina of the eye), and cause blindness.

MENINGITIS

Meningitis is an inflammation of the meninges (membranes surrounding the brain and spinal cord), resulting from viral or bacterial infection. It can strike at any age, but is more often seen in children. The viral variety is more common, but less serious. Untreated bacterial meningitis can result in coma or death.

Symptoms include an intense headache, followed by fever, vomiting, stiffness in the back and neck, and sensitivity to light. Diagnosis is usually made by lumbar puncture (inserting a fine needle into the lower back to draw a sample of spinal fluid). Analysis of this fluid will reveal whether the infection is bacterial, in which case it can be treated with antibiotics, or viral, in which case the treatment is more difficult. But full recovery is likely with rest and painkillers.

ENCEPHALITIS

This is a viral inflammation of the brain itself, which may be a result of common infections such as cold sores, glandular fever, measles or mumps. The symptoms are similar to those of meningitis: headache, fever and stiff or painful neck. However, encephalitis symptoms also include confusion and drowsiness, lack of co-ordination and fits, depending on which part of the brain is affected. Diagnosis is also made by lumbar puncture. Treatment consists of pain-killers and bed rest, and sometimes anti-epileptic drugs to prevent convulsions. Recovery is usually complete within a few weeks. Encephalitis can be fatal, but this is rare.

Danger Signals

Seek immediate medical advice if you notice these symptoms:

- A severe headache that strikes suddenly, without warning, or which intensifies dramatically.
- Sudden headache in someone previously headache-free.
- Sudden headaches striking someone with high blood pressure, heart disease or kidney problems.
- Headache following head injury and/or accompanied by nausea, dizziness, blurred vision, muscle weakness or personality changes.
- Any headache accompanied by seizures.
- Any headaches accompanied by fever – unless there is an obvious reason for the fever, like having the flu.
- Any decline in mental awareness or alertness (whether accompanied by headache or not).
- Headache accompanying localised pain in other parts of the body.
- Persistent headaches in children.
- Any headache that is aggravated by coughing, sneezing or stooping.
- Remember, if concerned in any way about any sort of headache – consult your doctor.

Helpful Addresses

There are a number of organisations that specialise in helping headache sufferers listed below. Most large NHS hospitals have pain clinics, to which your doctor can refer you.

British Migraine Association
178A High Road
West Byfleet
Surrey
KT14 7ED
(01932) 352468

The Migraine Trust
45 Great Ormond Street
London
WC1N 3HZ
(0171) 278 2676

Institute of Complementary Medicine
PO Box 194
London
SE16 1QZ
(0171) 636 9543

Medical Advisory Service
10 Barley Mow Passage
London
W4 3DY
(0181) 994 9874

The Pain Society
9 Bedford Square
London
WC1B 3RA
Send a stamped addressed envelope for their register of pain clinics.

Self-Help in Pain (SHIP)
33 Kingsdown Park
Tankerton
Kent
CT5 2DT
(01227) 264677

Migraine Diary

Migraines are often triggered by foods, situations or events. By filling in the diary, keeping track of your activities, food intake and stress levels, you should be able to build a picture of your migraine patterns.

DAY	FOOD	STRESS 1–10	CHANGE IN ROUTINE	ALLERGIES
1				
2				
3				
4				
5				
6				

DAY	FOOD	STRESS 1–10	CHANGE IN ROUTINE	ALLERGIES
7				
8				
9				
10				
11				
12				
13				
14				
15				
16				
17				
18				
19				

DAY	FOOD	STRESS 1–10	CHANGE IN ROUTINE	ALLERGIES
20				
21				
22				
23				
24				
25				
26				
27				
28				
29				
30				
31				